# MENTAL ILLNESS

## *LEARN THE EARLY SIGNS OF MENTAL ILLNESS IN TEENS*

**By Patricia A Carlisle**

# Introduction

I want to thank you and congratulate you for choosing the book, *"MENTAL ILLNESS: Learn The Early Signs of Mental Illness in Teens"*.

This book contains proven steps and strategies on how to become aware of the mental health signs in teens.

Mental illnesses in Teens are medical conditions that disrupt thinking, feeling, mood, ability to relate to others, and daily functioning. Mental illnesses can affect persons of any age, race, religion, or income. Mental illnesses are not the result of personal weakness, lack of character, or poor upbringing. Mental illness is an illness just like a physical illness.

It is becoming more and more apparent that mental illness in teens is a real issue that requires immediate attention. In a study conducted by the Center for Disease Control, it was revealed that up to 1 in 5 young people in the United States struggle with mental illness. It was also found that the prevalence of mental illness among America's youth seems to be increasing. Knowing the warning signs of mental illness has the potential to not just improve your child's life but in some cases save it.

Thanks again for choosing this book, I hope you enjoy it!

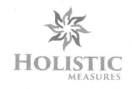

# ABOUT THE AUTHOR

## Patricia A. Carlisle, MSW, CBT

Patricia Carlisle- a Master Social Worker and Cognitive Behavioral Therapist (CBT) gives out an expression of how important it is for an individual to take into consideration the concept of self-assessment to know what human, technical and conceptual skills they posses to perform or to achieve what they desire, or to deal with everyday life. However, every particular group of people has their own unique set of ideas, traditions and events including the frame of mind according to which people perform but there are many who faces problems and fail to maintain a healthy mind set affecting their behaviors and performance to those around them.

People like Patricia Carlisle are among those who have felt this urge of serving people and helping them out of their mental crisis towards a healthy life. She has experienced some close encounters in her personal life regarding mental health issues in her family and friends that has encouraged her to pursue this as her career.

Currently Patricia Carlisle is serving as a Certified On-Line Cognitive Behavioral Therapist with an extensive 15years of experience using Cognitive-Behavior Therapy Techniques. She envisions a world where everyone gets mental health treatment with no mental health stigma and to make it real she has already set up her own Holistic Measure Online

Comprehensive Behavioral Healthcare Company after retiring from The Nord Center in The Partial Hospitalization Program (PHP) Dept for 5 years and Murtis H. Taylor Mental Health Center as a mental health counselor, psychological support technician and case manager for 10 years to emulsify her skills more professionally.

Along with this, she has wrote down her passion as a clinician in 25 or more short books to help individuals and families get their life back, freeing them of the restraints of negative thinking, anxiety and depression by using different approaches. She is highly appreciated among her clients for her flexibility and professionalism of dealing with them graciously. To reach her, make use of her direct website address: http://therapist2013.wix.com/e-therapy . As she is ready to inspire hope and contribute to health and well-being by providing the best online health care through comprehensive practice, education and research.

# TABLE OF CONTENT

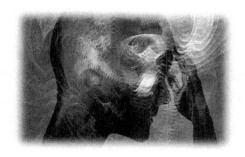

# Chapter 1

# EARLY SIGNS OF MENTAL ILLNESS IN TEENS

Mental health services and supports are available and the earlier you access them the better. Many teens live full lives with a mental health condition. More and more teens are speaking out about their experiences and connecting with others.

Teens aren't an easy time for parents, either. As Teens move through the various tumultuous transitions that accompany Teens physical, emotional, hormonal, sexual, social, intellectual-the pressures and problems they encounter can all too easily seem overwhelming. For many Teens, these and other pressures can lead to one or more of a variety of mental health disorders; all are matters of concern, and some are life-threatening.

## DISORDERS IN TEENS

Categories of diagnoses in these schemes may include mood disorders in Teens, anxiety disorders in Teens, psychotic disorders, eating disorders, developmental disorders, personality disorders, and many other categories. Commonly recognized categories of anxiety disorders include specific phobia, generalized anxiety disorder, Social Anxiety Disorder, Panic Disorder, Agoraphobia, Obsessive-Compulsive Disorder and Post-traumatic stress disorder in Teens.

# Chapter 2

# EARLY SYMPTOMS IN TEENS

Today, we classify mental illness in Teens based on the symptoms a person experiences and the clinical features of the illness, such as feeling hopeless or having delusions. But as we continue to gain a clearer understanding of how specific genes interact with illnesses or behaviors, we may be able to develop a much more sophisticated classification system that is directly linked to a biological cause of mental illness, rather than just symptoms.

For instance, some disorders in Teens have similar symptoms and clinical features but are actually very different in terms of their underlying biology. Thus, symptoms related to behavior or our mental lives clearly reflect variations or abnormalities in brain function.

Persons suffering from any of the severe mental disorders present with a variety of symptoms may include inappropriate anxiety, disturbances of thoughts and perception, and cognitive dysfunction. Often it is a good idea to first describe the symptoms and/or problems to your family physician or clergy.

Quite often the term mental illness in Teens conjures up pictures of dramatic madness or extreme cases of eccentricity, abnormal behavior and more. However, there are several subtle or border-line spectrum of mind or brain related illnesses that do not display such visible signs of mental illness.

While most mental disorders in Teens are known to show symptoms such as erratic, impulsive behavior either through talk mannerisms or actions, there are many disorders which are never displayed but are so subtle that many times the go unnoticed. Individuals, who have a known family history of mental disorders, will be able to recognize some of the signs and seek professional help to manage the disorder where necessary.

Besides, the signs or symptoms of illness in Teens are typically not the same for everybody and all ages. There are both cultural, social and ethnic variations, believe experts in the field of mental illness.

Further, as the reasons for occurrence of mental disorders are both a part of inherited genetic material as well as mutation of certain behavior-related physiologies, experts believe that with regular monitoring, review and constant alternative therapy, the signs of mental illness can be detected and effectively managed.

# Chapter 3

## SYMPTOMS OR SIGNS OF MENTAL ILLNESS

The earlier your child gets treatment, the more likely they are of overcoming and moving past their disorder. This is why it's extremely important that parents know the warning signs of mental illness in teens.

**From the American Psychiatric Foundation, common signs include:**

Decrease in school performance

Noticeable changes in sleeping/eating patterns

Continuous physical complaints

Acting out sexually

Prolonged negative attitude/mood

Alcohol/drug abuse

Threats or acts of self-harm

Frequent outbursts of anger

The typical signs of mental illness vary from adults to children:

Most pre-teenagers may become addicted to drugs or begin to use alcohol

A very significant feature is that performance in school is affected. Besides, there is a distinct fall in grades.

Inability to cope with daily problems and activities

There are changes in the sleeping as well as eating habits in these children

Pre-tanner's begin to complain repeatedly about physical problems

Continued attempts to over-ride authority; Show no desire to attend school; take to stealing to feed drug abuse.

Show symptoms of damaging property or destructive behavior

Are afraid of weight gain and do not know how to handle issues related to it.

Loss of appetite; continued negativity about every day issues and a strong tendency to commit suicide.

# Chapter 4

## THE SYMPTOMS IN TEENS VARIES DIFFERENTLY

Noticeable changes in activities and performance in school.

Though the child tries hard the grades continue to be poor.

There is display of worry and anxiety.

Children are prone to be Hyperactive in this stage.

There is higher incidence of nightmares and fear of darkness.

Demonstrates stubbornness to authority; does not agree with normal family or school rules. Increasingly become diffident. Disobedience as well as aggression increases.

Continues to throw or display dramatic scenes of temper, misbehavior, callousness as well as anger.

It has to be noted that behavior of this kind may eventually develop into full-fledged manifestation of mental disorders. The ability to identify the signs in the initial stages is critical for immediate and effective therapy.

Where medical science is quick to offer drug and pharma-based treatment the cure and solutions that these medicines provide are either temporary or short-term. Therefore, individuals who display the initial stages or signs of mental illness become dependent on drugs. The long-term implications of these are both physical as well as psychological.

Therefore, there is a need to explore other ways of dealing with the issue of mental illness that may be an alternate or non-medical therapy.

One such complementary form of wellness solution is based on a revolutionary natural phenomenon-The Trivedi Effect.

# Chapter 5

## THE TRIVEDI EFFECT

Before you begin to review the Trivedi Effect as an alternative or a complementary system for dealing with mental illness, here is brief introduction of the concept.

The Trivedi Effect is a natural phenomenon that when harnessed and transmitted by individuals, transforms living organisms and non-living material so they can function at a higher level and serve a greater purpose.

Tens of thousands of people throughout the world have experienced this phenomenon and are now enjoying the journey of their life.  Many of them have reported improvements such as:

Greater Mental clarity

Stronger relationships

Financial growth and prosperity

Higher quality sleep

Higher self confidence

Mental calm and inner peace

Better interpersonal relationships

Relief from Depression

Reduced anxiety and stress

Clearer perception

Greater Optimism

More Positive Mood

Improved ability to focus

Feeling of gratitude

Many people have even reported that the Trivedi Effect has transformed their relationships, dramatically increased their happiness and helped them discover their life's true purpose. Some benefits are experienced immediately, while others unfold over time. No matter how big or small the benefits seem to be, people everywhere have experienced remarkable and even life-changing results.

# Chapter 6

## GETTING TREATMENT

If you believe your son or daughter is struggling with a mental illness, it's important to seek out professional help. Many effective treatments and programs exist to help your family through this difficult time, but it can be hard finding the one that will do the most for your child.

Elevations RTC is a residential treatment center for adolescents struggling with issues, such as depression, anxiety, ADHD, and many more. We can help lead your child back onto a healthier path.

Treatment may include psychotherapy (individual, family, group), skills programs (learning, social skills, behavior), and psychiatric medication, and be provided in a variety of inpatient, outpatient, or day treatment settings. This may include special schools, residential placements, hospitals, private offices, or community clinics.

Psychotherapy and psychiatric medication are two major treatment options, as well as supportive interventions. Most people diagnosed with a serious mental illness can experience relief from their symptoms by actively participating in an individual treatment plan.

Without treatment the consequences of mental illness for the individual and society are staggering, unnecessary disability, homelessness, inappropriate incarceration, suicide and wasted lives; the economic cost of untreated mental illness is more than 100 billion dollars each years in the United States.

Early identification and treatment is of vital importance; by ensuring access to the treatment and recovery supports that are proven effective, recovery is accelerated and the further harm related to the course of illness is minimized.

# Chapter 7

# KEY TIPS FOR PARENTS

**Keep communication constant, open, and honest:**
Your children should not only know that they can talk to you
about anything, you have to be committed to introduce topics
of concern and do so openly. Talk about your own experiences
and fears when you were an adolescent. Let them know that
they are not alone; nor are their anxieties unique.

**Understand that mental health disorders are
treatable:** Arm yourself with information about the most
common mental health disorders among adolescents; speak
with your child's pediatrician, your local health department,
your religious leader, and your child's school representatives
about what sorts of information are available from them.

Be attentive to your teen's behavior: Adolescence is indeed, a
time of transition and change, but severe, dramatic, or abrupt
changes in behavior can be a strong indicators of serious
mental health issues.

**Mental health "Red Flags" Parents Should Be Alert
For:**

Excessive sleeping, beyond usual teenage fatigue, which could
indicate depression or substance abuse; difficulty in sleeping,
insomnia, and other sleep disorders

Loss of self-esteem

Abandonment or loss of interest in favorite pastimes

Unexpected and dramatic decline in academic performance

Weight loss and loss of appetite, which could indicate an eating disorder

Personality shifts and changes, such as aggressiveness and excess anger that are sharply out of character and could indicate psychological, drug, or sexual problem

# Chapter 8

# KEY MENTAL HEALTH ISSUES IN TEENS

**Depression in Teens:**  While all of us are subject to "the blues," clinical depression is a serious medical condition requiring immediate treatment.  Watch for:

Changes in sleep patterns

Unexpected weeping or excessive moodiness

Eating habits that result in noticeable weight loss or gain

Expressions of hopelessness or worthlessness

Paranoia and excessive secrecy

Self-mutilation or mention of hurting himself or herself

Obsessive body-image concerns

Excessive isolation

Abandonment of friends and social groups

**Eating disorders in Teens:**  Body image concerns can become obsessions, resulting in starting weight loss, severely affecting the adolescent's health.

**Anorexia:**  Avoidance of food and noticeable changes in eating habits should trigger concern.

**Bulimia:**  Purging (forced vomiting) after eating-alert for both dramatic weight loss without changes in eating habits (which could, of course, indicate other health issues that require a doctor's attention) and also for immediate trips to the bathroom or other private spot after a meal.

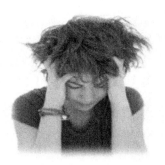

## Chapter 9

## SIGNS YOUR TEEN NEEDS MENTAL HEALTH TREATMENT

Teens go through emotional ups and downs all the time. Hormones are changing, life can seem overwhelming, and without much life experience, a young adult can feel misguided. When parents are busy working, or a natural separation from family occurs, teens may turn to friends instead of parents.

Peer support can be helpful for certain issues. But when the symptoms of a mental illness are present, more than a good friend is needed. The problem is, teens may not understand what the feelings they experience mean. As a parent it's important to stay connected so that you notice any changes or any symptoms of a mental illness in your child. Mental illness includes depression; anxiety; bipolar disorder; schizophrenia; borderline personality disorder; post-traumatic stress disorder (PTSD); attention-deficit disorder (ADD); attention-deficit hyperactivity disorder (ADHD) and many more disorders that can interfere with your teen's daily life.

In an effort to self-medicate to control the symptoms of the undiagnosed and untreated mental illness-teens without help may turn to drugs, alcohol, or eating disorders to feel better, to escape, to numb out, or to feel in control.

**Below are some ways to tell if your teen may need mental health treatment:**

**Mood swings:** How can you decipher a moody teen from a true set of mood swings that indicate mental illness? You know your child better than anyone else. Trust that you can recognize a shift in mood that is out of character for your son or daughter.

**Behavioral changes:** The same thing goes for your child's behavior. Of course behavioral choices changes as your teen gets older, but if your son or daughter is presenting as a different person to you, this may indicate a mental illness or substance abuse.

**Consequences in school and among friends:** A mental illness can distract from concentration, which can affect school performance and the ability to sustain relationships with peers.

**Physical symptoms:** Decreased energy, changes in eating and sleeping, frequent stomachaches, headaches, and backaches, and neglect of personal appearance and hygiene (such as showering less often and not keeping up on grooming) can be signs that mental health treatment is needed.

**Self-medicating:** If you find any indicators of drug or alcohol use, self-harm, and eating disorder, or other forms of escape, the link to mental illness may be direct. An effort to make oneself feel better can show a great need for mental health treatment.

If you see any of these signs, seek help for your child. With appropriate assessment, identification, and intervention, all mental illnesses can be treated and managed.

# Chapter 10

# HOW TO TALK TO TEENS ABOUT MENTAL ILLNESS

Most kids form together a working knowledge of mental health topics through bits and pieces gathered from their peers, parents and the media, the National Alliance of Mental Illness, a nationwide grassroots nonprofit that provides treatment support and advocacy for the mentally ill.  However, this body of information is often inaccurate.

Kids should know more about the stereotypes for [mental illness] than what it actually is, who serves as the youth program director of NAMI's Montgomery County, Maryland, chapter. "They don't really know the symptoms.  They don't really know what the person goes through."

There are many misconceptions about mental illness, that all people with mental illness are violent; that psychiatric diseases are moral or character flaws; and that those who have them can't live normal lives.  In reality, the majorities are nonviolent, and coping methods ranging from medication and therapy to exercise can help individuals stay healthy and productive.

**Find a Teaching Opportunity:**  "It can be helpful to bring [mental illness] up in context-for example, if your child knows that someone is having difficulties with their mood or behavior and his questions about it.  As mental illness becomes less stigmatized, we are also hearing more about people in the news with mental illness.  This can be a good opportunity to start a discussion.  As with any more serious discussion, choosing a time when you and your child can focus is helpful, such as over a meal, in a long car ride or during a quiet time at home.

But you don't necessarily need to use a news peg or a media moment as an excuse to raise the subject. A discussion about mental illness, she emphasizes, is "a conversation that anyone can have. It shouldn't be like a 'birds and the bees' type of talk.

**Tailor Your Language to Different Age Group:** When speaking to your child or adolescent about mental illness, it's important to keep in mind their age and developmental level. For preschool children, keep it simple. With this age, you may only need to have these discussions if someone they know is affected. School-aged children may have more questions. With this age, it's helpful to be clear, simple and direct and to follow their lead in terms of how much information you give them.

With teenagers, you can be more specific-especially because their age group faces a high risk of depression and suicide. Teaching them the names and traits of various illnesses gives them the knowledge and coping skills they need if they, or someone they know, experiences a psychiatric disorder firsthand. That way, they can seek support from a teacher, a parent or a counselor.

**Tell Them They Have a Safety Net:** Since mental illness is fairly common-with as many as 61 percent of people experiencing a well-specified psychiatric disorder by age 12, children may first learn about it through personal experience. In this case, they're usually advised to confide in a trusted adult. But a fear of stigma often keeps them from coming forward. "A lot of the time, [kids] believe if they have a mental illness, nobody should know, they think people will look at them differently.

# Conclusion

Thank you again for choosing this book!

I hope this book was able to help you to identify with different types of mental health issues your teen may be facing.

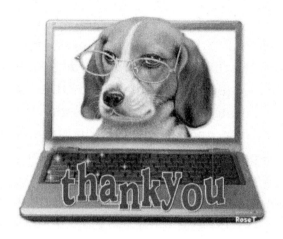

Finally, if you enjoyed this book, would you be kind enough to leave a review for this book on Amazon? It'd be greatly appreciated!

Thank you and good luck!

# Preview Of 'HOW TO LIVE WITH PEOPLE AFFECTED WITH MENTAL ILLNESS'

## Chapter 1: INTRODUCTION

Stigma associated with mental illness and psychiatric treatment, and the discrimination towards people with mental illnesses that frequently results from this, are the main obstacles preventing early and successful treatment. To reduce such stigma and discrimination towards mentally ill people and especially those with schizophrenia, the World Psychiatric Association's (WPA) anti stigma programmed 'Open the Doors' is currently being implemented in more than 20 countries. The programmed has been undertaken in seven project centers in Germany. Public information programs and education measures aimed at selected target groups are intended to improve the public's knowledge regarding symptomatolgy, causes and treatment options for schizophrenia. Improved knowledge should in turn reduce prejudice and negative education. Protest and contact are the key elements of anti stigma strategies recommended by the WPA and various research groups. These anti stigma strategies include improving psychiatric care and psycho-education of patients and families, involving patients and family members in all anti stigma activities, including anti stigma education in the training of health care providers, initiating education activities in the general public and specific target groups, and promoting social and legal action to reduce discrimination.

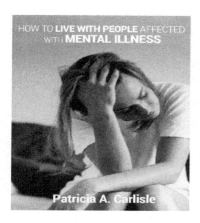

# How to live with people affected with mental illness.

# Check Out My Other Books

Below you'll find some of my other popular books that are popular on Amazon and Kindle as well. Alternatively, you can visit my author page on Amazon to see other work done by me. (https://amazon.com/author/patriciacarlisle)

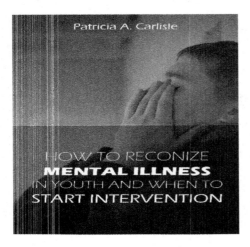

**How to Recognize Mental Illness in Youth and When to Start Intervention.**

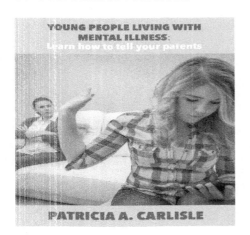

**YOUNG PEOPLE LIVING WITH MENTAL ILLNESS: LEARN HOW TO TELL YOUR PARENTS.**

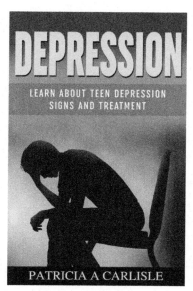

**DEPRESSION: Learn About Teen Depression Signs and Treatment.**

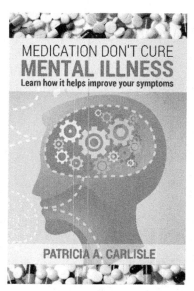

**MEDICATION DON'T CURE MENTAL ILLNESS: Learn how it helps improve your symptoms.**

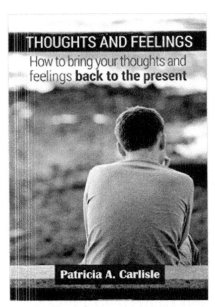

**THOUGHTS AND FEELINGS: How to Bring Your Thoughts and Feelings Back to the Present.**

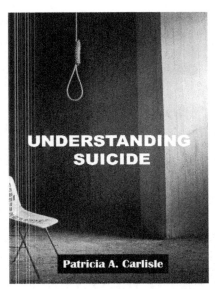

**Understanding Suicide.**

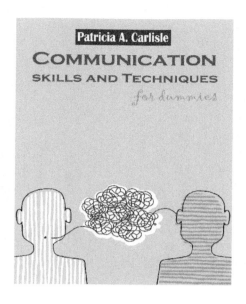

**COMMUNICATION SKILLS AND TECHNIQUES FOR DUMMIES.**

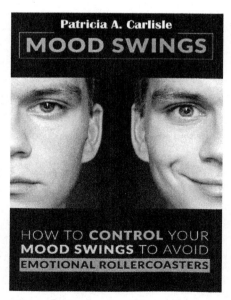

**Mood Swings: How to control your mood swings to avoid emotional rollercoster's.**

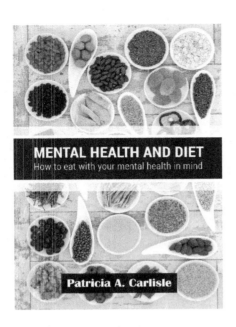

**Mental Health and diet: How to eat with your mental health in mind.**

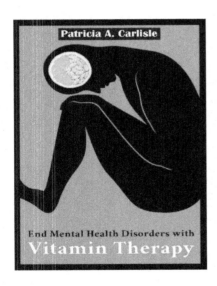

**End Mental Disorders with vitamin therapy.**

## BONUS: FREE BEGINNERS GUIDE TO YOGA & MEDITATION

"Stressed out? Do You Feel like The World Is Crashing Down Around You? Want To Take A Vacation That Will Relax Your Mind, Body And Spirit? Well this Easy to Read Step By Step E-Book Makes It all Possible!"

# What cat you learn from this book?

The different styles of yoga

Basic positions of yoga

# How to maximize your "workout" space

Meditation for health and wellness ridding yourself of tension headaches with yoga

How to do a yoga workout at your desk

And so much more!

So many people have achieved a sense of wellness they have never felt before just through a few short yoga sessions.

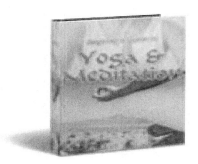

**YOU CAN GET THIS E-BOOK IN THE BACK OF ANY OF MY KINDLE BOOKS**

# NOTES

# NOTES

# NOTES